The Weight Loss Blueprint

Building a Strong Mindset for Lasting Results

Stephanie C. Levine

Copyright

Table Of Content

- Final Thoughts

- Next Steps

Introduction

Welcome to "The Weight Loss Blueprint: Building a Strong Mindset for Lasting Results." I'm thrilled to embark on this journey with you towards achieving your health and wellness goals. In this book, we will delve deep into the psychology of weight loss, emphasizing the power of mindset in attaining sustainable results.

The purpose of this book is to equip you with the tools, knowledge, and strategies necessary to cultivate a resilient mindset that will support you throughout your weight loss journey. By understanding the fundamental principles of mindset and implementing practical techniques, you will not only shed excess pounds but also develop a healthier relationship with food, exercise, and yourself.

Get ready to challenge old habits, overcome obstacles, and embrace a new way of thinking that empowers you to achieve lasting transformation. Let's embark on this transformative journey together and pave the way for a healthier, happier you.

Chapter 1
Understanding Weight Loss

In this chapter, we will delve deep into the fundamental aspects of weight loss. By understanding the concepts of weight loss, defining clear goals, dispelling common misconceptions, and exploring the science behind them, you will lay a solid foundation for your journey toward a healthier lifestyle.

1. **Defining Weight Loss Goals**:

Setting clear and achievable goals is crucial for any successful weight loss journey. Start by defining your specific objectives, whether it's shedding a certain number of pounds, fitting into a particular clothing size, or improving overall health markers like blood pressure or cholesterol levels. SMART is for Specific, Measurable, Achievable, Relevant, and Time-bound. This is how you should set your goals. For example, instead of saying "I want to lose weight," specify how much weight you aim to lose within a certain timeframe, such as "I aim to lose 10 pounds in the next two months." This clarity will provide you with a roadmap and motivation to stay on track.

2. **Common Misconceptions**:

There are numerous misconceptions surrounding weight loss, which often lead to frustration and disappointment. Let's address some of these myths:

A. Rapid Weight Loss is Sustainable: Many people believe that crash diets or extreme exercise regimens will lead to long-term weight loss. However, these methods often result in muscle loss, metabolic slowdown, and rebound weight gain once the diet ends. Sustainable weight loss requires gradual, healthy lifestyle changes.

B. Carbohydrates are the Enemy: Carbohydrates are often vilified in popular diets, leading many to believe that cutting carbohydrates is essential for weight loss. While reducing refined carbs and sugars can be beneficial, complex carbohydrates like whole

grains, fruits, and vegetables are essential for
providing energy and essential nutrients.

C. Skipping Meals Leads to Weight Loss:

Some believe that skipping meals, especially breakfast, can accelerate weight loss by reducing calorie intake. However, skipping meals can lead to overeating later in the day, lower energy levels, and disrupted metabolism. Regular, balanced meals are crucial for sustainable weight loss.

D. Spot Reduction is Possible:

Many people believe that targeting specific areas of the body through exercises like crunches or thigh workouts will reduce fat in those areas. However, spot reduction is a myth. Weight loss occurs systematically throughout the body, influenced by factors like genetics and overall body composition.

E. All Calories are Equal:

One prevalent misconception is that all calories are the same, regardless of their source. While it's true that calories measure energy, the body metabolizes different types of calories differently. For example, calories from protein, carbohydrates, and fats have varying effects on hunger, metabolism, and satiety. Focusing solely on calorie counting without considering nutrient quality can hinder weight loss efforts and overall health.

F. Supplements Guarantee Weight Loss:

Many people believe that taking weight loss supplements or fat-burning pills is a quick fix for shedding excess pounds. However, most of these products are not regulated by the FDA and lack scientific evidence supporting their effectiveness and safety. Furthermore, relying on supplements without making lifestyle changes is unlikely to lead to sustainable weight loss. It's essential to prioritize a balanced diet and regular exercise over-relying on supplements alone.

G. You Must Avoid Fat to Lose Weight: The low-fat diet trend of the past has left many people fearing dietary fat, believing it to be the culprit behind weight gain. However, not all fats are created equal, and certain types of fats, such as monounsaturated and polyunsaturated fats found in avocados, nuts, and olive oil, are essential for overall health and can even support weight loss by promoting satiety and aiding nutrient absorption. Rather than demonizing all fats, focus on incorporating healthy fats in moderation as part of a balanced diet.

3. The Science Behind Weight Loss:

Understanding the physiological processes involved in weight loss can demystify the journey and empower you to make informed decisions. Weight loss primarily occurs when the body expends more calories than it consumes, creating a calorie deficit. This deficit can be achieved through a combination of dietary changes (reducing calorie intake) and increased physical activity (burning calories). Moreover, factors such as metabolism, hormonal balance, and genetics play significant roles in individual weight loss experiences. For instance, some people may have a naturally higher metabolism, allowing them to burn calories more efficiently, while others may struggle with hormonal imbalances that affect appetite and fat storage.

Furthermore, sustainable weight loss encompasses more than just calorie counting. It involves adopting a balanced diet rich in whole foods, incorporating regular physical activity, managing stress levels, prioritizing adequate sleep, and cultivating a positive mindset.

By understanding these principles and dispelling common myths, you can embark on your weight loss journey with confidence and clarity, laying the groundwork for lasting results.In this chapter, we have explored the fundamental aspects of weight loss, including setting clear goals, debunking common misconceptions, and understanding the scientific principles behind it.

Armed with this knowledge, you are now better equipped to navigate your journey towards a healthier, happier you. In the following chapters, we will delve deeper into practical strategies and techniques to help you achieve your weight loss goals sustainably and effectively.

Chapter 2
Building a Strong Mindset

In the journey toward achieving your weight loss goals, building a strong mindset is fundamental. This chapter will delve into the significance of mindset in weight loss, strategies for overcoming mental barriers, and practical tips for cultivating positive habits that support your long-term success.

1. **Importance of Mindset in Weight Loss:**

Your mindset plays a pivotal role in your ability to achieve and maintain weight loss. It shapes your beliefs, attitudes, and behaviors toward food, exercise, and overall health. This is the reason it's so important to develop a good mindset:

A. Mindset Drives Behavior:

Your thoughts influence your actions. A positive mindset can lead to healthier choices, such as opting for nutritious foods and engaging in regular physical activity.

B. Resilience:

Weight loss is often accompanied by challenges and setbacks. A strong mindset enables you to bounce back from setbacks, stay motivated, and persevere despite obstacles.

C. Long-Term Success:

Temporary diets may yield short-term results, but sustaining weight loss requires a shift in mindset. Developing a sustainable approach fosters lasting habits that support your health and well-being over time.

D. Self-Efficacy:

A positive mindset enhances your belief in your ability to succeed, known as self-efficacy. When you believe in yourself and your capacity to make meaningful changes, you're more likely to persist in the face of challenges and setbacks. Self-efficacy empowers you to take proactive steps toward your weight loss goals and maintain confidence in your ability to overcome obstacles along the way.

E. Shift in Perspective:

Cultivating a strong mindset involves shifting your perspective on weight loss from a short-term fix to a long-term lifestyle change. Instead of focusing solely on the number on the scale, you begin to prioritize overall health and well-being. This shift in perspective encourages sustainable habits and fosters a more balanced relationship with food, exercise, and self-care. By viewing weight loss as part of a holistic approach to health, you're more likely to embrace habits that support lasting results and prioritize your overall wellness journey.

2. Overcoming Mental Barriers:

Achieving lasting weight loss requires addressing and overcoming mental barriers that may impede progress. Here are common mental hurdles and strategies to overcome them:

A. Negative Self-Talk:

Positive affirmations should be used to counter negative thinking. Accept yourself, be kind to yourself, and put progress ahead of perfection.

B. Fear of Failure:

Embrace setbacks as learning opportunities rather than viewing them as failures. Set realistic goals, celebrate small victories, and cultivate resilience in the face of challenges.

C. Emotional Eating:

Recognize triggers for emotional eating, such as stress or boredom, and develop alternative coping mechanisms, such as mindfulness or journaling. If required, call friends, family, or a therapist for helping hands.

D. All-or-Nothing Thinking:

Avoid rigid, black-and-white thinking about food and exercise. Embrace flexibility and moderation, allowing yourself to enjoy occasional treats while maintaining overall balance.

E. Negative Body Image:

Addressing negative body image perceptions can be a significant barrier to weight loss. Practice self-acceptance and focus on appreciating your body for its strength and resilience. Challenge unrealistic beauty standards and shift your focus from appearance-based goals to health and vitality. Engage in activities that promote body positivity, such as yoga or meditation, and surround yourself with supportive individuals who value you for more than just your physical appearance.

F. Perfectionism:

Striving for perfection can lead to feelings of frustration and discouragement when progress doesn't meet unrealistic expectations. Instead of aiming for perfection, embrace progress over perfectionism. Acknowledge that obstacles are a normal part of the path and rejoice in little wins. Focus on continuous improvement rather than striving for flawless outcomes. Adopting a growth mindset allows you to learn from challenges and adapt your approach to better support your long-term goals.

G. Social Pressures and Temptations:

Social situations and external pressures can pose challenges to your weight loss efforts. Whether it's peer pressure to indulge in unhealthy foods or feeling isolated due to dietary restrictions,

navigating social environments can be daunting.
Develop strategies to cope with social pressures,
such as communicating your goals with friends
and family, seeking out supportive social circles,
or bringing nutritious snacks to social
gatherings. Practice assertiveness in setting
boundaries and prioritize your health and well-
being, even in social settings. Remember that
your health is a personal priority, and it's okay to
advocate for yourself and make choices that
align with your goals.

3. Cultivating Positive Habits:

Building a strong mindset involves cultivating
positive habits that support your weight loss
journey. Here are strategies to foster healthy
habits:

A. Goal Setting:

Set specific, measurable, achievable, relevant, and time-bound (SMART) goals to guide your progress. Break larger goals into smaller milestones to track your success along the way.

B. Consistency:

Establish a consistent routine for meals, exercise, and self-care practices. Consistency builds momentum and reinforces healthy habits over time.

C. Self-Care:

Prioritize self-care activities that nourish your body, mind, and spirit. This includes adequate sleep, stress management techniques, and activities that bring you joy and fulfillment.

D. Mindful Eating:

Practice mindful eating by paying attention to hunger and fullness cues, savoring each bite, and eating with intention rather than on autopilot.

E. Support System:

Surround yourself with a supportive network of friends, family, or online communities who encourage and motivate you on your journey.

By focusing on cultivating a strong mindset, overcoming mental barriers, and nurturing positive habits, you can set yourself up for lasting success in your weight loss endeavors. Remember that transformation takes time and effort, but with dedication and perseverance, you can achieve your goals and embrace a healthier, happier lifestyle.

Chapter 3
Setting the Foundation

In this chapter, we will delve into the crucial steps of setting a strong foundation for your weight loss journey. By assessing your current habits and lifestyle, setting effective goals, and creating a realistic plan, you will lay the groundwork for sustainable and lasting results.

1. **Assessing Current Habits and Lifestyle:**

Before embarking on any weight loss journey, it's essential to take stock of your current habits and lifestyle. This self-assessment provides valuable insights into what factors contribute to your current weight, health, and overall well-being. Here's how to approach it:

A. **Food Intake:**

Keep a food diary for at least a week to track what you eat and drink. Note portion sizes, meal times, and any emotional triggers that influence your eating habits.

B. **Physical Activity:**

Evaluate your current level of physical activity. How often do you exercise? What types of activities do you enjoy? Are there any barriers preventing you from being more active?

C. **Sleep Patterns:**

Assess your sleep quality and quantity. Do you get enough restful sleep each night? Are there any sleep disturbances or patterns that may affect your weight loss efforts?

D. **Stress Levels:**

Identify sources of stress in your life and how they impact your eating and exercise habits. Stress eating and lack of motivation are common responses to stressors.

E. **Social Support:**

Consider your support system. Do you have friends, family, or online communities that can offer encouragement and accountability on your journey?

2. Goal Setting Techniques

Setting clear and achievable goals is paramount to success in weight loss. Here are some techniques to help you set effective goals:

A. SMART Goals:

Make your goals Specific, Measurable, Achievable, Relevant, and Time-bound. For example, A SMART goal would be, "I will lose 10 pounds in the next two months by exercising four times a week and reducing my daily calorie intake by 500 calories,"

B. Long-term vs. Short-term Goals:

Break down your overarching weight loss goal into smaller, manageable milestones. Celebrating these smaller victories will keep you motivated along the way.

C. Focus on Behavior Changes:

Shift your focus from outcome-based goals (like reaching a certain weight) to behavior-based goals (such as eating more vegetables or exercising regularly). This approach promotes sustainable lifestyle changes rather than quick fixes.

D. Write Them Down:

Document your goals in a journal or on a vision board where you can see them daily. This visual reminder will help keep you focused and accountable.

3. Creating a Realistic Plan

With your goals in mind, it's time to devise a realistic plan that aligns with your lifestyle and preferences:

A. **Nutrition Plan:**

Based on your food diary and goals, create a balanced and nutritious meal plan. Be cautious of portion sizes, mindful eating practices, and full foods.

B. **Exercise Routine:**

Design an exercise routine that includes activities you enjoy and can commit to regularly. Make an effort to include strength, flexibility, and cardiovascular conditioning in your regimen.

C. **Schedule and Prioritize:**

Block out time in your schedule for meal prep, workouts, and self-care activities. Give these appointments your whole attention, just as you would any other responsibility.

D. **Anticipate Challenges:**

Identify potential obstacles that may derail your progress, such as cravings, social events, or time constraints.Make action plans to proactively overcome these challenges.

E. Seek Support:

Share your plan with friends, family, or a professional coach who can offer encouragement, accountability, and guidance along the way.

By diligently assessing your current habits, setting SMART goals, and creating a realistic plan, you'll lay a solid foundation for your weight loss journey. Stay committed, stay resilient, and remember that progress takes time and persistence.

Chapter 4
Nutrition Essentials

In this chapter, we delve into the foundational aspects of nutrition essential for successful weight loss. Understanding macronutrients, mastering meal planning, and portion control, and adopting healthy eating strategies are key components of building a strong mindset for lasting results.

1. Understanding Macronutrients

Macronutrients are essential nutrients required by the body in large quantities to provide energy, support growth, and maintain overall health. There are three primary macronutrients: carbohydrates, proteins, and fats. Each macronutrient serves a distinct role in the body's functioning and contributes to various physiological processes. Balancing macronutrient intake is crucial for achieving optimal health and supporting specific goals such as weight management, muscle building, and athletic performance.

A. Proteins:

Proteins are essential for muscle repair and growth, satiety, and overall metabolic function. Sources include lean meats, poultry, fish, tofu, legumes, and dairy products. Aim to include a source of protein in every meal to support muscle preservation during weight loss.

B. Carbohydrates:

Carbohydrates provide energy for daily activities and exercise. Focus on complex carbohydrates like whole grains, fruits, vegetables, and legumes, which offer fiber for satiety and sustained energy levels. Limit refined carbohydrates such as white bread, sugary snacks, and processed foods, as they can spike blood sugar levels and lead to cravings.

C. Fats:

Healthy fats are crucial for hormone production, brain function, and nutrient absorption. Add unsaturated fat-containing foods to your diet, such as avocados, nuts, seeds, olive oil, and fatty fish like mackerel and salmon. While fats are more calorie-dense, they contribute to feeling satisfied after meals and can aid in weight loss when consumed in moderation.

2. Meal Planning and Portion Control:

A. **Set Goals**:

Begin by setting realistic goals based on your calorie needs and weight loss objectives. Use online calculators or consult with a nutritionist to determine your daily calorie target for weight loss.

B. **Meal Prep:**

Dedicate time each week to plan and prepare meals in advance. This not only saves time but also ensures you have healthy options readily available, reducing the temptation to indulge in convenient yet calorie-dense foods.

C. Balanced Meals:

Aim for balanced meals that include a source of protein, complex carbohydrates, and healthy fats. Incorporate a variety of colorful fruits and vegetables to maximize nutrient intake and promote satiety.

D. Portion Control:

Use measuring tools or visual cues to control portion sizes. Pay attention to recommended serving sizes and avoid mindless eating, especially when dining out or snacking.

E. Mindful Eating:

Eat consciously by taking your time, chewing your food well, and observing your body's signals of fullness and hunger. This encourages a healthier connection with food and helps avoid overindulging.

3. Healthy Eating Strategies:

A. Hydration:

Stay hydrated by drinking plenty of water throughout the day. Sometimes humans misunderstand their thirst for hunger, which leads to excessive chewing. Try to drink eight glasses of water or more if it's hot outside or you're physically engaged.

B. Smart Snacking:

Choose nutrient-dense snacks like fruits, vegetables, yogurt, nuts, or whole-grain crackers. Avoid processed snacks high in added sugars and unhealthy fats, which can sabotage your weight loss efforts.

C. **Reading Labels**:

Develop the habit of reading food labels to make informed choices about the products you consume. Pay attention to serving sizes, calorie content, and ingredient lists, opting for options with minimal additives and preservatives.

D. **Seek Support:**

Surround yourself with a supportive community of friends, family, or online forums dedicated to healthy living. Having accountability partners can help you stay motivated, share tips and recipes, and celebrate milestones along your weight loss journey.

By understanding macronutrients, mastering
meal planning, and portion control, and adopting
healthy eating strategies, you lay the foundation
for sustainable weight loss and cultivate a strong
mindset for lasting results. Remember,
consistency and patience are key, and every
small step towards healthier eating habits brings
you closer to your goals.

Chapter 5
Exercise and Movement

In this chapter, we delve into the essential role of exercise and movement in achieving lasting weight loss results. We'll explore how to design an effective exercise routine, how to incorporate physical activity into daily life, and strategies for overcoming exercise plateaus.

1. Designing an Effective Exercise Routine:

Designing an effective exercise routine is crucial for achieving weight loss goals. Here are the key steps to create a routine that works for you:

A. Establish Specific Goals:

Begin by outlining your fitness goals.Do you want to lose weight, build muscle, or improve overall health? Setting clear, achievable goals will guide your exercise routine.

B. Assess Your Current Fitness Level:

Understand your current fitness level to determine where to begin. Consider factors like cardiovascular endurance, strength, flexibility, and any physical limitations.

C. Choose the Right Activities:

Select exercises that align with your goals and preferences.This could involve a combination of strength training (lifting weights, bodyweight exercises) and aerobic workouts (running, cycling, etc.).

D. Create a Balanced Routine:

Ensure your routine includes a balance of cardiovascular, strength, and flexibility exercises. Incorporating variety will prevent boredom and help target different muscle groups.

E. Gradually Increase Intensity:

Start with manageable intensity levels and gradually increase as your fitness improves. This progressive approach prevents injuries and keeps your body challenged.

F. Schedule Regular Workouts:

Consistency is key to success. Schedule workouts at times that fit your lifestyle and stick to your plan as much as possible.

2. Incorporating Physical Activity into Daily Life:

In addition to structured exercise, integrating physical activity into your daily life can boost calorie burn and support weight loss efforts. Here's how to incorporate more movement into your routine:

A. Take Active Breaks:

Instead of sitting for long periods, take short breaks to stretch, walk, or do simple exercises. Even a few minutes of activity can add up throughout the day.

B. Walk Whenever Possible:

Opt for walking or cycling instead of driving short distances. Use stairs instead of elevators, and aim to walk whenever feasible.

C. Multitask with Exercise:

Combine exercise with other activities, such as listening to podcasts while walking or doing bodyweight exercises while watching TV.

D. **Engage in Recreational Activities**:

Find enjoyable physical activities like dancing, hiking, or playing sports that don't feel like traditional exercise but still keep you moving.

3. Overcoming Exercise Plateaus:

Plateaus are common in fitness journeys, but they can be overcome with the right approach. Here's how to push past exercise plateaus:

A. Adjust Your Routine:

If you've hit a plateau, it may be time to change up your exercise routine. Try new activities, increase intensity, or incorporate different types of workouts to challenge your body in new ways.

B. Focus on Progressive Overload:

Gradually increase the intensity, duration, or frequency of your workouts to continually challenge your body and stimulate progress.

C. Monitor Your Progress:

Keep track of your workouts, progress, and any changes in your body composition. This will help you identify patterns and make informed adjustments to your routine.

D. Prioritize Recovery:

Ensure you're allowing enough time for rest and recovery between workouts. Adequate rest is essential for muscle repair and growth, which can prevent burnout and support long-term progress.

E. Seek Support:

Consider working with a personal trainer or fitness coach who can provide guidance, accountability, and personalized strategies to help you overcome plateaus.

By following these strategies for designing an effective exercise routine, incorporating physical activity into daily life, and overcoming exercise plateaus, you'll build a strong foundation for lasting weight loss success. Remember, consistency, patience, and perseverance are key on your journey to a healthier lifestyle.

Chapter 6
Managing Stress and Emotional Eating

In this chapter, we will delve into the critical aspects of managing stress and emotional eating to build a strong mindset for lasting weight loss results. We will explore techniques to identify triggers, effective stress management strategies, and mindful eating practices that can aid in your journey toward a healthier lifestyle.

1. Identifying Triggers:

A. Understanding Emotional Eating:

Emotional eating is a common response to stress, anxiety, boredom, or even happiness. It involves consuming food not out of hunger but to cope with emotions. To tackle emotional eating effectively, it's essential to identify the triggers that lead to it.

The things that trigger different people can include:

- Stressful situations at work or home
- Relationship issues
- Loneliness or boredom
- Negative self-talk
- Unpleasant emotions such as sadness, anger, or anxiety

B. Keeping a Trigger Journal:

Keeping a trigger journal can be immensely helpful in identifying patterns and understanding the root causes of emotional eating. In this journal, note down:

- When you feel the urge to eat emotionally
- The feelings you were feeling at the time.
- The situations or things that set off those feelings

2. Stress Management Techniques:

A. Deep Breathing Exercises:

Exercises involving deep breathing can ease tension and encourage calm. By taking a deep inhale via your nose, letting your belly expand, then gently exhaling through your mouth, you can practice diaphragmatic breathing. Every time you feel anxious or overwhelmed, repeat this for a little while.

B. Progressive Muscle Relaxation (PMR):

PMR entails methodically tensing and relaxing each of your body's muscular groups. Ascending to your head from your toes, concentrate on each muscle group for a brief period of time before letting go of the tension. This method can facilitate the discharge of physical and mental tension, promoting a sense of calmness.

C. Mindfulness Meditation:

During mindfulness meditation, you focus on the here and now while letting go of any judgment. Choose a calm area, choose a comfortable seat, and concentrate on your breathing or a particular object. Bring your feelings back to what is happening at the moment when they stray.

Frequent practice helps lower stress levels and raise self-awareness.

D. Guided Imagery:

Using your imagination to conjure up serene and tranquil mental images is known as guided imagery. Locate a quiet area, close your eyes, and picture yourself in a peaceful setting, such a forest or beach. As you let yourself go completely into relaxation, concentrate on the sights, sounds, and sensations of this imagined location.

E. Physical Activity:

Regular physical activity might be a useful strategy for lowering stress and elevating mood. Whatever your activity of choice—yoga, the gym, or a brisk walk—find something you enjoy doing and incorporate it into your daily schedule. Exercise can give pent-up stress and tension a much-needed release and aid in the release of endorphins, which are naturally occurring mood enhancers.

F. Journaling:

Journaling is a therapeutic practice that allows you to express your thoughts, feelings, and concerns on paper. Set aside a few minutes each day to write freely about your emotions, experiences, and any stressors you may be facing. Journaling can help you gain clarity, process your emotions, and find constructive ways to cope with stress.

3. Mindful Eating Practices:

A. Eating Without Distractions:

Avoid eating while watching TV, scrolling through your phone, or working. Instead, create a peaceful eating environment free from distractions. Pay attention to the flavors, textures, and sensations of each bite.

B. Listen to Your Body:

Practice intuitive eating by tuning in to your body's hunger and fullness cues. Eat when you're physically hungry and stop when you're satisfied, even if there's food left on your plate. Learning to distinguish between physical hunger and emotional hunger is key to overcoming emotional eating.

C. Savor Each Bite:

Take your time to chew each bite thoroughly and savor the flavors of your food. Eating slowly allows your brain to register feelings of fullness, reducing the likelihood of overeating. Engage all your senses while eating to fully appreciate the experience.

D. Gratitude Practice:

Before each meal, take a moment to express gratitude for the food in front of you. Reflect on the journey of the food from its source to your plate, acknowledging the effort and resources involved in its production. Cultivating a sense of gratitude can enhance your appreciation for the nourishment provided by each meal and promote mindful eating.

E. Portion Awareness:

Practice portion control by paying attention to the size of your servings. Use smaller plates and utensils to help regulate portion sizes and prevent overeating. Before serving yourself, take a moment to assess your hunger levels and portion out a reasonable amount of food. Eat slowly and mindfully, savoring each bite, and stop when you feel comfortably satisfied.

F. **Engage Your Senses**:

Fully engage your senses while eating to enhance the sensory experience of each meal. Notice the colors, textures, and aromas of your food before taking a bite. Chew slowly and pay attention to the flavors and sensations as you eat. Take breaks between bites to appreciate the interplay of flavors and the satisfaction that comes from nourishing your body. By engaging all your senses, you can elevate the enjoyment of eating and foster a deeper connection with your food.

By implementing the techniques outlined in this chapter, you can effectively manage stress, overcome emotional eating, and cultivate a mindful approach to eating. Remember that building a strong mindset for lasting weight loss results is a journey that requires patience, self-compassion, and consistent practice. You can reach your wellness and health objectives if you put in the necessary effort and persistence.

Chapter 7
Sleep and Recovery

In your journey towards achieving your weight loss goals, one of the most crucial yet often overlooked aspects is sleep and recovery. In this chapter, we'll delve into the importance of sleep in weight loss, strategies to improve sleep quality, and recovery techniques for optimal results.

1. Importance of Sleep in Weight Loss:

Sleep is not just a period of rest; it plays a fundamental role in your body's ability to regulate metabolism, control hunger hormones, and repair tissues. Here's why sleep matters in your weight loss journey:

A. Metabolism Regulation:

Quality sleep is essential for regulating metabolism. When you're sleep-deprived, your body's ability to process and utilize nutrients efficiently decreases, which can lead to weight gain.

B. Hormonal Balance:

Sleep deprivation disrupts the balance of hunger hormones, ghrelin, and leptin. Ghrelin stimulates appetite, while leptin signals satiety. Lack of sleep increases ghrelin levels and decreases leptin levels, leading to increased appetite and cravings for high-calorie foods.

C. **Energy Levels:**

Adequate sleep ensures optimal energy levels throughout the day, which is crucial for maintaining an active lifestyle and sticking to your exercise routine.

D. **Muscle Recovery**:

During sleep, your body undergoes repair and recovery processes, including muscle tissue repair. Quality sleep is essential for muscle recovery and growth, especially if you're engaging in strength training exercises as part of your weight loss regimen.

2. **Improving Sleep Quality:**

Now that we understand the importance of sleep in weight loss, let's explore strategies to enhance sleep quality:

A. **Create a Regular Sleep Schedule**: Even on the weekends, try to get to bed and wake up at the same time every day. This enhances the quality of your sleep and aids your body's internal clock.

B. **Create a Relaxing Bedtime Routine:** Develop pre-sleep rituals such as reading, taking a warm bath, or practicing relaxation techniques like deep breathing or meditation to signal to your body that it's time to wind down.

C. **Optimize Your Sleep Environment:**

Make sure your bedroom is cold, quiet, and dark to promote good sleep. Invest on pillows that help your sleeping posture and a comfy mattress.

D. Limit Exposure to Screens:

The blue light emitted by electronic devices can interfere with your body's natural sleep-wake cycle. Avoid using smartphones, tablets, and computers at least an hour before bedtime.

E. Watch Your Caffeine Intake:

Limit consumption of caffeine, especially in the afternoon and evening, as it can disrupt sleep patterns and make it harder to fall asleep.

3. Recovery Strategies for Optimal Results:

In addition to prioritizing quality sleep, incorporating recovery strategies into your routine can enhance your weight loss efforts:

A. **Active Recovery:**

Engage in low-intensity activities such as walking, yoga, or swimming on rest days to promote blood flow, reduce muscle soreness, and aid in recovery.

B. **Proper Nutrition:**

Fuel your body with nutrient-dense foods that support recovery, such as lean proteins, complex carbohydrates, and healthy fats. Regular hydration is also vital for the best possible recuperation.

C. Foam Rolling and Stretching:

Incorporate foam rolling and stretching exercises into your post-workout routine to alleviate muscle tension, improve flexibility, and enhance recovery.

D. Quality Sleep Supplements:

Consider incorporating natural sleep aids such as melatonin, magnesium, or valerian root under the guidance of a healthcare professional to improve sleep quality if needed.

E. Mindfulness and Stress Management:

Practice mindfulness techniques such as meditation, journaling, or progressive muscle relaxation to reduce stress levels, promote relaxation, and improve sleep quality.

By prioritizing quality sleep and implementing effective recovery strategies, you'll not only enhance your weight loss journey but also promote overall health and well-being. Remember, building a strong mindset for lasting results begins with taking care of your body's fundamental needs, including sleep and recovery.

Chapter 8
Staying Motivated and Consistent

In the journey towards weight loss, maintaining motivation and consistency are key components for achieving lasting results. In this chapter, we will delve into the strategies for finding and sustaining motivation, overcoming setbacks, and celebrating achievements along the way.

1. Finding Your Motivation:

A. Identify Your Why:

Start by understanding why you want to lose weight. Is it for health reasons, to improve self-confidence, or to lead a more active lifestyle? Write down your reasons and keep them visible as constant reminders.

B. Set Specific Goals:

Create clear, achievable goals that align with your motivations. Whether it's losing a certain amount of weight, fitting into a specific clothing size, or improving fitness levels, having tangible targets can keep you focused.

C. Visualize Success:

Imagine yourself at your desired weight, feeling healthier and happier. Visualizing your success can reinforce your commitment and help overcome moments of doubt.

D. **Find Inspirational Sources**:

Surround yourself with sources of inspiration, such as success stories, motivational quotes. Engage with supportive communities or seek guidance from a mentor or coach.

E. **Track Your Progress:**

Keep track of your achievements, no matter how small. Whether it's recording workouts, measuring inches lost, or noting improvements in energy levels, tracking progress can boost motivation by showing tangible results.

2. **Overcoming Setbacks:**

A. **Expect Challenges:**

Understand that setbacks are a natural part of any journey, including weight loss. Anticipating challenges can help you prepare mentally and emotionally to deal with them effectively.

B. Learn from Setbacks:

Instead of dwelling on setbacks, view them as opportunities for growth. Analyze what triggered the setback and identify strategies to overcome similar obstacles in the future.

C. Stay Flexible:

Be willing to adapt your approach if certain strategies are not yielding the desired results. Flexibility is essential for navigating obstacles and finding alternative solutions.

D. Seek Support:

Reach out to friends, family, or support groups during challenging times. Sharing your struggles with others can provide encouragement, perspective, and accountability.

E. Practice Self-Compassion:

Be kind to yourself when facing setbacks. Avoid self-criticism and negative self-talk, and instead, focus on treating yourself with understanding, forgiveness, and encouragement.

3. Celebrating Achievements:

A. Acknowledge Milestones:

Take time to celebrate your progress and achievements along the way. Whether it's reaching a weight loss milestone, mastering a new exercise, or adopting healthier habits, acknowledge and reward yourself for your efforts.

B. Reflect on Success:

Reflect on how far you've come since starting your weight loss journey. Recognize the changes you've made, both physically and mentally, and appreciate the hard work and dedication it took to get there.

C. Share Your Success:

Share your achievements with others who have supported you throughout your journey. Whether it's through social media, a personal blog, or in-person conversations, sharing your success can inspire others and reinforce your commitment.

D. Set New Goals:

After celebrating your achievements, set new goals to continue progressing towards your ultimate vision of health and wellness. Having new challenges to strive for can maintain momentum and keep you motivated.

E. Practice Gratitude:

Cultivate gratitude for the progress you've made and the opportunities you have to pursue your goals. Expressing gratitude can shift your focus from what you lack to what you have accomplished, fostering a positive mindset for continued success.

Staying motivated and consistent on your weight loss journey requires dedication, resilience, and a supportive mindset. By finding your motivation, overcoming setbacks, and celebrating achievements, you can build a strong foundation for lasting results and a healthier lifestyle. Understand that each step you take will get you one step closer to what you want to achieve.

Conclusion

In wrapping up "The Weight Loss Blueprint:
Building a Strong Mindset for Lasting Results,"
it's essential to reflect on the journey we've
embarked on together and to provide guidance
on what comes next.

Final Thoughts:

Throughout this book, we've explored the
critical role of mindset in achieving sustainable
weight loss. We've discussed the importance of
shifting our perspective from short-term fixes to
long-term habits and behaviors. By cultivating a
strong mindset, rooted in self-awareness,
positivity, and resilience, we lay the foundation

for lasting change. Remember, every setback is an opportunity for growth, and every small victory is a step toward our ultimate goal. Celebrate your accomplishments, accept the process, and treat yourself with kindness as you go.

Next Steps:

As you close this book, consider the following steps to continue your journey towards a healthier lifestyle:

A. **Set Clear Goals**:

Take some time to reassess your weight loss goals and break them down into manageable, achievable steps.To maintain motivation and focus, put them in writing and go over them frequently.

B. Develop a Routine:

Establish a consistent routine that includes regular exercise, balanced nutrition, adequate sleep, and stress management techniques.To create enduring habits, one must be consistent.

C. Stay Accountable:

Whether it's through a supportive friend, a coach, or an online community, find someone or something to hold you accountable to your goals. Share your progress, setbacks, and successes with others who understand and support your journey.

D. Practice Self-Compassion:

Be kind to yourself, especially when faced with challenges or setbacks. Remember that change takes time, and perfection is not the goal. You should be kind and compassionate to yourself just as you would a friend.

E. Celebrate Progress:

No matter how tiny, recognize and celebrate your accomplishments. Recognize the effort you've put in and the progress you've made towards a healthier lifestyle.

F. Stay Educated:

Continue to educate yourself about nutrition, exercise, and mindfulness techniques. Knowledge is power, and the more you understand about your body and mind, the better equipped you'll be to make informed decisions and stay on track.

G. Stay Inspired:

Surround yourself with sources of inspiration, whether it's motivational quotes, success stories, or role models who inspire you to be your best self. Draw strength and inspiration from those who have overcome similar challenges and remember that you are capable of achieving your goals.

Remember, the journey to sustainable weight loss is not always easy, but with the right mindset, support, and determination, you have the power to transform your health and well-being for the better. Keep believing in yourself, stay committed to your goals, and never underestimate the strength of your own mindset. You've got this!